How to Break Bad Habits and Create Great Ones

By

Kurt Francis

Rick Morris
2018

Copyright © 2018 by Kurt Francis

First Printing: 2018

ISBN: 978-0-9963197-2-0

Cronus Media Ventures, LLC
Columbus, OH 43004

www.CronusMediaVentures.com

Dedication

I want to dedicate this book to Fernando Francis. He has believed in me and supported me. He has been so continually positive day after day. He has shown me his discipline and willpower. I have never witnessed any human being on this planet who operated on a level like he has. He would rise early just after 5 AM and head to work. 14 hours later, he would arrive home. I would sometimes "time him" after he walked in that door from is long day at work. Most days, it would be 53 second to just over 60 seconds and he would be at his desk studying and preparing for his class the next day. This happened day after day for over 2 years. He was studying in his second language as well. If we want to talk about dedication, let me talk about Fernando.

I also dedicate this book to my mom Ione, my father Vivian, my sister Karen, and my brothers Charl and Rory.

Thank you for helping me to understand what it takes to break habits and create and form new habits.

Contents

Acknowledgements

We are where we are in life because of others. The older I get, the more I realize this. I want to acknowledge and give thanks to the people who have molded my spirit and attitude. I want to acknowledge those who have given me grace when I never deserved it – hose who were kind to me even after I had messed up so badly.

I acknowledge my father and mother, Vivian and Ione Francis, who relentlessly and unconditionally loved me when I had failed them.

When I never believed in myself, or faced challenges that seemed impossible to bear, my mother was there. When my faith ran out, my mother's faith and belief kicked in. She believed in me when I did not believe in myself. My parents taught me discipline and willpower from an early age. My father taught me discipline through watching him. I don't know of a 20-year-old who could keep up with my dad when he was over 75 years of age. He would work a full day as a civil engineer, in heat that was around 35 degrees Celsius (95 degrees F) at the age of 75 years without an air conditioner in his office, then go home and run 20 km or ride 50 km to train for the World Championship Ironman in Kona, Hawaii. The discipline that it takes for anyone at any age to train for an Ironman – a swim of 2.4 miles (3.8 km), bike ride of 112 miles (180 km), then run of 26 miles (42 km which is a full marathon) – under any condition is remarkable. No 20-year-old has ever won one, by the way. Yes, my father is my hero.

My mother and father taught me the power of a habit. They taught me this book! I acknowledge them in every way I can.

My sister, Karen Francis Cunningham, who loved me even when she did not understand my life. She has always gone out of her way and gone the extra mile for me. There is no one that I have ever met who has cared for so many people like she has. From driving her students home because their parents who were too inebriated to pick their children up from school to driving 862 kilometers (535 miles) and then back to care for her ex-mother-in-law, she has taught me to care for people no matter the cost. As a school teacher she did not earn a lot, yet she always found money to care for people. Some would criticize her for wasting gasoline driving to people to help them; she never let that bother her. Oh, may I say, I was one who had judged her in the past. How I have had to humble myself.

I have this most incredible brother Charl. He has selflessly given his life to serve others. I have never experienced anyone who serves people the way he has. From his own children to our parents to myself. Many years ago when I was going through a rough time in my life, a time where I could hardly talk about it, he brought humor to me. He caused me to laugh so hard. I will never forget that moment. He has played a massive role in my life and taught me how to serve other people: my friends, my partner, my customers, my clients. If there is anyone who understands serving at a high level with "high touch," it is Charl. This planet still has a lot to learn from him. I know of some politicians who could learn a lot from him.

My youngest brother Rory, what a gift he has been. We all remember the day he was born. From that day, he has been a delight to all of us. I remember when he was a little boy, he had weaved this basket. He learnt that at his school that he attended. There were 11 children in the school. I remember my mother had guests staying over. When the guests were about to leave, he gave away this basket that he made that was really precious. I said to him, "You don't have to give it away." This small and young little boy said to me, "I have to give it away." He has always been a giver. He has given his life away to others. The way he gives to his children and his wife has been a massive example to this planet. Always friendly, kind and giving.

There are others I would like to mention:

Chuck and Leigh Jackson who gave me a home when I moved to the United States of America. I will never ever forget their love.

Ed Delph and his wife Becky, who sponsored me to come to the United States of America and afforded me this opportunity. I will always be grateful and acknowledge them. They put their necks out and supported me.

David Romero, who was the CEO of the company I have worked for longer than any other company. He believed in me and always gave me grace and support no matter the mistakes I made. He has been a mentor and a coach who put my interest before his or the company's interest. He taught me the meaning of leadership. He treated me like family and made me part of his family. I will be eternally thankful for his belief in me.

Sara Jackson, my direct supervisor, boss and friend who gave me the freedom to share things with her without me feeling insecure.

Would you like you more of Kurt in your life? He would love to hear from you!

Connect with Kurt:

Kurt@KurtFrancis.com

www.KurtFrancis.com

www.epochinvigoration.com

Foreword

In the 17 years I have been in the real estate industry, I have seen my share of speakers, coaches, and snake oil salesmen. I've been to more conferences and seminars than I can count. In all that time, only a few people stand out in my memory as influential and remarkable. Kurt Francis is one of those people!

I first met Kurt in 2015 at a national sales meeting for the home warranty company with whom I was employed. He was asked to address our sales force as a motivational element in our conference. To say he succeeded would be an understatement. Despite the fact that he had just returned from out of the country and had a full-blown case of the flu, Kurt delivered a rousing presentation ending in thunderous applause. It was definitely the highlight of my trip.

Imagine how honored and surprised I was when I received a Facebook friend request a few months later from Kurt. Someone like THAT wanted to connect with ME? Kurt stated that he felt we were destined to know one another and to do great things. Here I am, three years later, writing the foreword to his book! I guess he knew what he was talking about.

I also had the honor of completing Kurt's coaching program called My Epoch Challenge. If you truly want a life-altering, inspiring experience, I highly recommend it. Much of this book comes from a portion of that coaching program, and it leaves you wanting more and asking, "What's next?"
No doubt, many of us have heard the statistic that it takes 21 days to form a new habit. I know I certainly never questioned it. Then along comes this guy to tell me that to truly change the course of my life by shifting my behavior, it takes 99 days. I'll admit I was skeptical.

I have been a student of behavior and personal motivations my entire adult life. I guess it comes from being in sales. I am fascinated by what compels people to do what they do, even if it is destructive or at odds with their own self-interest. As Kurt would say, "Why do you do that horrible thing to you?" The short answer is, habits.

As human beings, we get stuck in a pattern of behavior. Even if we know it's bad, the pattern is comfortable, even addictive. It can take a great deal of pressure to change course and abandon our comfort zone. That is where Kurt shines. His matter-of-fact nature allows him to call shenanigans on our pathetic excuses for not changing our behavior.

Kurt's background of life in Apartheid South Africa brings a unique color and perspective to his work. Kurt and I have spoken at length about his respect for Nelson Mandela and everything Mandela went through to help his people. If Mandela could do all that, surely I can change a small behavior to make my life better in some way. Better yet, I can help improve the lives of others.

What I love most about Kurt is his passion, drive, and energy. He is genuinely motivated to help others become better than they are and to reach their goals. Kurt is also very purposeful in all he does. Take this book, for example. It has exactly 99 pages. That is no accident. The number 99 happens to be quite important to central premise surrounding habit formation. Kurt doesn't do things by mistake.

Kurt Francis is truly one of the most inspiring people I have ever met. I am so lucky to have his friendship, guidance, and encouragement in my life. He sincerely wants everyone to live their best lives possible. His passion is apparent in everything he does, including this book. I hope you enjoy reading it as much as I did and that it helps make your life just a bit better than it was before you read it!

Stephen Meadows

Coach/Trainer/Sales Professional/Consultant

Author of the books *Meet More Make More, I've Got My Own Problems,* and *Brand Yourself Online in 30 Days*

Columbus, Ohio

September, 2018

Wowcome!

Wowcome to your "Transvigoration™". Wowcome to you breaking through barriers, limits and boundaries that you have never achieved before.

Are you sick and tired of not experiencing a breakthrough in breaking bad habits?

Are you agitated and frustrated at not overcoming that habit that is holding you back in:

- your career
- your income
- your spiritual life
- your mental state
- your emotions
- your physical body
- your dreams and goals
- your wealth
- your family
- your friends
- your coworkers

and even your spouse or better half? Have you gotten to a place of despair and zero hope of ever overcoming obstacles?

Are you agonizing over the thought of never breaking through a bad habit?

Are you feeling worthless about your life achievement so far and just don't know how to break through?

Do you feel like your life is like you are at an airport departure lounge and you are seeing everyone else get on their flights and reach their destinations but you are stuck in the terminal, not even knowing what flight is going to take you?

Are you feeling like you have no future, like an aircraft that has been sent to the desert "boneyard" to retire and just waste away?

Wowcome. Wowcome. Wowcome.

Why a Wowcome? When one breaks barriers, limitations, boundaries and bad habits, we become wowed even at ourselves. How many times have we made New Year's resolutions and entered the new year with great hope and by the end of January we are back where we were? All the energy and emotions that you put into your New Year's resolutions and then ending up not just back where you were, but worse off than you were.

Wowcome to saying goodbye to some of the pain, agony, discomfort, frustration, hopelessness, depression, lack of vision, unbelief and sadness you have had in your life.

Wowcome to you appreciating yourself more. Wowcome to you loving yourself more. Wowcome to you wanting to help others more. Wowcome to you believing in yourself. Wowcome to you in believing in others. Wowcome to you believing in your spouse. Wowcome to you believing in your family, your kids, your parents, your brothers and sisters. Wowcome to believing in your co-workers. Wowcome to you believing in your passion.

Now is not the time to get tired of the word Wowcome … too many have got sick of the "Wowcome" and they lost the wowcome … they lost the wow out of their life. Their careers, their jobs, their families have lost the WOW. Their kids, parents and spouses have lost the wow … Marriages have lost the wow … Their dreams have lost the wow. Everything about them has lost the wow.

I read this quote on *someecards.com*: "*Marriage is like a deck of cards. In the beginning all you need is two hearts and a diamond. By the end, you wish you had a club and a spade* ... OK, that was a joke ... My parents have been married for 57 years and they still have the wow. Not all marriages end up that way.

Do you remember when you wanted a specific job or wanted to work for a certain company and

> *Your wowcomes are going to cause you some phenomenal outcomes.*

you got it and you wanted to shout and smile and spin around with joy? Every emotion possible took control of your face. You wanted to put it on Facebook, and every social media site you could find ... Do you remember how you went out that night to rejoice and celebrate when you got that job? And, how is it now? Have you still got that Wow? It was a wow ... so many lose the wow ... You are going to get hungry for that wow again ... This is not just a little welcome...it is a wowcome ... You're going to start waking up in the mornings every day with a wowcome ... Your face is going to want it!!!!

For you to have phenomenal outcomes, you're going to have to have some phenomenal wowcomes. You're going to have to wowcome some breaking bad habits and wave goodbye to them. You are going to have to wowcome some great new habits that are going to take you to the life you have wanted and the life that you can have. You're going to have to wowcome yourself to some changes in your life.

Wowcome to a different kind of thinking. Wowcome to not expecting yourself to be perfect. Wowcome to not judging others and expecting them to be perfect. You are about to witness some imperfections in my English ... my grammar, my spelling ... It is being written the way I speak ... I speak with an accent and that is not all ... I write with an accent ... I spell with an accent ... I think with an accent ... I dream with an accent ... I live with an accent ... and by the way, so do you. You have got an accent ... and I like your accent ... I dreamt for years as a little boy that I would have an accent like yours ... When you live your life with your "accent," you going be you ... You are going to have some breakthroughs.

We all think differently; we all speak differently!!!! Yes, you have an accent ... YES, YOU SPEAK FUNNY; YES, YOU THINK FUNNY; YES, YOU DREAM FUNNY ... Yes, you are different!!!! Yes, you are unique. Yes, you were created that way. I am created that way. Get over it. You are beautiful just as you are. Your life is filled with wonderful gifts, talents and skills. Others are different and that is OK. So let's not judge them nor criticize them ... ouch. I have done that so many times and 1,000 times more than you have.

I used to live on the 29th floor in downtown San Diego. Just about every day getting into the elevator I would greet people and someone would ask me where am I from ... I would say ... from San Diego ... and I could see them look at me like "ahhhhhh no he is not from San Diego ... he has an accent." So I would say to them, Oh, do you mean my accent? Yes, they reply, oh ... I got my accent at NORDSTROM for $1,000 and I can take it back to them without a receipt. I continue to tell them that I am originally from South Africa for 5 generations so that makes me an official African American Without a Tan. Wowcome to you wanting to grow.

Wowcome to you wanting to break some bad habits and replace them with great habits.

A Harvard Medical School study calculated 20 to 40% of cancer cases and 50% of cancer deaths could be prevented by one's input and output specifically if people quit smoking, avoided heavy drinking, kept a healthy weight and got just 30 minutes of moderate exercise. It all comes down to breaking bad habits and forming new great habits.

What is a habit? How would you define it? A habit is a repeated behavior and has a tendency to reoccur non-consciously. The smallest little behavior, if repeated enough times will become habit without much effort. Most actions repeated enough times become steadfast habits that are often difficult to break.

Wowcome to your habit breaking and creating awareness.

"Ninety-nine percent of the failures come from people who have the habit of making excuses." – George Washington Carver

Chapter 1: Ground Zero

We often use the term "Ground Zero." After 9/11, it became a word that many used. Like many words we use, they originally had another meaning. I remember when my grandmother grew up in South Africa, the word "gay" did not refer to sexual orientation but rather an emotional state of being happy, joyful, carefree. In the 1890s the word was used to describe optimism and being optimistic. People would call it the Gay Nineties (1890). In 1941, Warner Brothers produced a short film called *The Gay Parisian* which related to free expression of emotional and ideology. We have all experienced many words that their meanings have changed by societies and cultures.

Ground Zero is certainly one of them. Initially, "Ground Zero" was meant to describe the point directly above, below, or at which a nuclear explosion occurs. Some may use the term as the epicenter of a disaster or explosion. The world started using it to describe the exact location of the World Trade Center after the 9/11 attacks. Many people have become very unhappy with our culture giving "Ground Zero" new meaning. Anyone who was alive and old enough to comprehend the day that the twin towers and the Pentagon were hit by aircrafts as well as the flight UA93 which crashed in a field in Pennsylvania, will be able to describe what ground zero was. The world was stuck to their televisions and became familiar with the term.

More recently, we are seeing our culture take the term "Ground Zero" a step further and describe it as when an individual's emotional, physical or psychological state sinks so low that they hit rock bottom.

I am certainly not saying that anyone who desires to break a bad habit, and replace it with a healthy and uplifting habit, needs to hit rock bottom first. Often when people do hit their rock bottom, breaking habits can seem easier.

I believe your Ground Zero can be where you realize that the pain you are going through is no longer tolerable or acceptable or you have reached a place where you no longer are willing to tolerate that emotional, psychological, physical, financial or relationship state. It is a point where you say enough is enough. With every bad habit there is some pain. The pain is manifested in either physical, emotional, financial or worst of all, relationship hardships. Certain drugs at the time may be really pleasant, yet devastating to other areas of our lives.

My question to you is where is your Ground Zero or what is your Ground Zero? What bad habit are you wanting to break? Let me ask you this, what actions and behaviors are limiting your potential of being the person you want to be or that you can be? Where is there unnecessary resistance in your life that is causing you above-normal stress?

As one gets older, we get used to stress and we tolerate more stress than a younger person. Some may say, well, we tolerate it more because we have become callous. Callus is an area of skin that is hard. Calluses are formed at certain points that have received repeated rubbing over a period of time. The skin hardens from continued pressure or resistance. Calluses are formed for a purpose, and that is to protect our feet or hands. One of my brothers, Charl, is a phenomenal musician. When he plays his guitar and sings he captivates an audience every time. His unique style and voice always draws fans. Only the few who know him, know how many hours upon hours he practices. His fingers from practicing his guitar became callous and so hard. Obviously his calluses protect his

> *To find our "Ground Zero," we sometimes have to go through the calluses in our life.*

fingers. If I started playing guitar and practiced the same amount of hours he does, well, my fingers would be bleeding very soon and probably get infected.

Our emotions, physiological and physical (including action) state all become callous after years of putting pressure or stress on any part of our life. Our actions and habits become callous. We are all habitual beings. Everyone has habits and more habits than we realize.

Habits are the number one reason of us becoming "callous." The continued repetitive actions we take cause us to get hard. Our actions get hard. Our physical body gets hard. Our emotions get hard. Our thought process gets hard and we become stubborn and we become callous. The callus protects us. So breaking a habit is breaking the callus that protects us. We live in a bubble of protection. Our whole life is a callus.

When deciding what bad habit you want to break, first look at the Ground Zero, where does the explosion need to happen. What outcome do I want to Wowcome? When we know the outcome, we will know what we need to wowcome.

Did you know that 91% of New Year's resolutions never materialize successfully? According to Statistical Brain Research Institute, only 9.2% of people felt they were successful in achieving their resolutions. Huffington Post quoted a statistic that only 8% of people actually keep their New Year's resolutions.

The only few good reasons to have New Year's resolutions are:
1. To create a conversation starter with someone you are interested in
2. To have a good laugh at others
3. To find out which of your friends do actually want to improve themselves, they just don't know how

4. To find out what you don't like about yourself and that you are desperately crying out for someone to help you … well, not really.

Actually, there are statistics that people who do make New Year's resolutions do end up working toward improving themselves and tend to be more conscious of it. Also, people who make New Year's resolutions tend to be more positive and optimistic in life and see the glass full and over flowing even if there is nothing inside the glass. These people are often happier than others who see the glass as half empty.

What is your Ground Zero? What "explosion" do you need to happen in your life?

"We are what we repeatedly do. Excellence, then, is not an act, but a habit."
– Will Durant

Chapter 2: Six Mistakes

We turn our lives around not only by breaking bad habits but breaking habits that are not adding value to our lives and then by replacing these bad and unwanted habits with great habits that will build our lives.

The 6 big mistakes to avoid when breaking a habit are closely related to why people fail at being and feeling successful at their New Year's resolutions.

Mistake #1: Focus on the Bad Habit

The first mistake to avoid when breaking a bad or unwanted habit is to keep focusing on the habit you want to break. What you focus on, expands. When something expands, it demands more attention. By expanding and when something demands more attention, the picture in your mind gets bigger. The bigger the picture gets, the more you tend to visualize it. The more you visualize it and think about it, your brain treats it like those massive photographic printers at Costco that print out hundreds of photographs. Your brain keeps on reproducing this picture and you end up with 1,000s of pictures in your mind. The more you think about it, the more you desire it. Pornography works the same way. What your mind sees, your mind desires.

Mistake #2: The Soul Tie

What your mind desires, you start making an emotional connection to. Your emotions are directly related to your thoughts. Remember that we make decisions based upon logic but we act on emotions. So when our emotions get connected to a habit, we start acting upon it. The more we think about the undesirable habit, the more emotions we attach to it and the bigger the emotion, the bigger the action. Emotions equal motion. It becomes a soul tie. We actually have to break the soul tie. A soul tie is an emotional tie. The more we think about it, the more we see it. The more we see it, the greater the emotional soul tie. The law of attraction is powerful. We attract certain emotions and desires just by seeing and thinking.

Mistake #3: Talking About the Bad Habit

Your tongue is a powerful weapon. Your tongue can take you to your destiny, goal and dream. Your tongue can divide goodness from destruction. We become the things we talk about. The more you talk about a habit, the more it will take control. You gotta change the way you speak. Just cut it out and stop it. The more you speak about it, the more you focus on it. As I mentioned, the more you focus on anything, the more it expands. When something expands, it demands more attention. You just have to stop it. If you catch yourself saying anything about it, practice the antidote which is the words "Just Stop It." Like Nike taught us "Just Do It," you need to "Just Stop It." Just stop talking about it. It is like vomit coming out of your mouth. You're breaking a habit, for crying out loud, then Just Stop talking about it. Every time you talk about it, imagine vomit coming out of your mouth.

I was visiting a friend in Atlanta in November 2009 for Thanksgiving. Saturday morning, November 28th, was one of the most embarrassing days of my life. I had eaten something the night before and had some alcohol that did not quite agree with me or I did not agree with it. The next morning this friend took me to a great restaurant for brunch. The restaurant's decor, ambiance, setting were great. I ordered some coffee soon after we sat down. I then ordered their special Eggs Benedict. Within a minute of receiving it – I had not even tasted it yet – I suddenly felt terribly ill. Within seconds of feeling ill, I vomited all over the table, I mean ALL over the table. It was like a massive fountain with tremendous force. I was shocked, surprised and could not believe what had just happened. Nor could anyone else in that restaurant believe what they had just witnessed. Others watched and seemed surprised as I was. I have never ever felt so embarrassed in my entire life. I was speechless. I did not know where to look. It was the most humiliating experience ever. The view looked terrible. The table looked gross. The faces of people looked even more crazy. It smelt nasty. There was nothing nice about it. The friend of mine, remained calm and collected and he said something really nice and funny and even made me laugh in the midst of the situation. He still reminds me of it and he loves bringing it up. Well, now I laugh about it and I do not mind bringing it up. I can assure you, it is better bringing it up now than bringing it up then on the table!

When you are breaking a habit and you keep on speaking about it, all you are doing is vomiting. Vomiting, vomiting and vomiting. Shut up, you ugly thing! Yes, you are not ugly because of the outside, you are ugly because of the inside. It is what comes out of you that is really nasty, ugly. That food looked good when it came in to me, but sure did not look good coming out of me. When you keep on speaking about the bad habit, you look nasty, sound nasty and smell nasty. Everything is nasty about it.

Mistake #4: Hanging Out with the Same People

During the time I ran my first "My Epoch Challenge," my life began to expand. This is a 99-day program that "transvigorates™" one's life and brings alignment of all of the 8 areas of one's life. During this online course I decided to provide a session on "The 6 Steps of How to Upgrade Your Relationships." Never did I ever realize how this would impact my life. This will be one of the next books I will be writing. Dr. David McClelland, a social psychologist from Harvard who did more than

30 years of research on human behavior, contributed motivational Need Theory. He also developed new scoring systems for the Thematic Apperception Tests, known as TAT. One thing he said that really captivated my attention, *"95% of our failures or our successes have to do with the people we associate ourselves with."* When I first read that, I thought that was ridiculous. The more I studied it and thought about it, the more I believed it. Now I teach it because I have experienced it.

I started putting this principle in action and wow, my life has changed. I immediately made a decision that I was going to upgrade my relationships. Wow. We become the people we hang out and associate with. We start eating what they eat. We start drinking what they drink. We start dressing like them. We start talking like them, sounding like them, thinking like them, acting (behaving) like them, using words like them. We start producing like them. We start earning like them. We start driving cars like them. We start believing like them. We even start sharing similar political views like them. We start sharing similar social views like them. We start living in neighborhoods like them. Jim Rohn said "You're the average of the five people you spend the most time with." You are the combined average of their life styles, health, wealth and income.

If you are serious about breaking a habit, stop hanging out with the people that are doing the things you no longer want to be doing. Some of them may be extended family. It may be neighbors, co-workers, cousins, old school and college friends you have to reconsider. Anyone who encourages you to keep on doing what they are doing and it is not in line with the habits you are wanting to break, then leave them. It may be temporary. It may be forever. It depends on the habit and depends on the people. Every situation is different.

If you are flying an aircraft, and the radar tells you that there are vicious storms ahead, the wise thing is for the pilot to avoid them. You are the pilot of your life. You are the captain. You make the decision. If you are flying and there is heavy fog and heavy moisture in the air and the avoidance system is telling you "Terrain, Terrain, Terrain." Terrain does not mean there is a lot of rain, it means terrain. Terrain is not some actress's name. It means, there is an object coming up close and you as a pilot need to pull up on the yoke and increase power and lift. It means do it now. It means take action. It means respond. This is not the time to speak to the co-pilot and first officer and say, well let's pray, let's have a prayer meeting. No. It means, full power and pick up the freaken yoke now and get lift. It does not mean sit back and look out the window. Take action and go above the obstacle, terrain, hindrance or anything that will stop your flight path. If people are in your flight path, go to a higher altitude. If you work for a company and the people who are part of the company are people you need to avoid, you may have to leave.

If people are in your flight path, go to a higher altitude.

Years ago in South Africa every Easter weekend from Thursday evening until Monday lunch time 150 young adults (19 years old to 35 years old) would go away. The weekends would be a time for fun, relationship building, teaching and growth for young adults. There was great music with live musicians, great sound and good accommodations. I was asked to lead the camps but declined for about 3 years until one specific year I felt strongly to do so. The year I agreed I had a vision to impact many younger adults' lives. There was already a committee of young adults who'd run the camps for a few years. My vision was to take the camp to over 600 people. To make the camps more motivational and really invigorate them in every area of their life, I decided I would change the name of the camp from Encounter camp to "Break Thru" camp. There were many changes I wanted to make, for example, when the buses arrived on Thursday evening, I did not want anyone to stand in line to register. I know how people hate standing in lines. I wanted them to have a great experience from the minute they arrived. I told the "Wowcome" committee that I wanted more registration tables. "OK," they said, "we will have 2 tables and not just 1." I said what, no, I want 12 tables with 3 people at each table." Well, I had opposition. There was someone on the leadership who was a handbrake for me. Every single thing, from changing the name of the camp to all the small changes, he would fight to keep everything the same. He said "if you change the name of the camp, no one would come." Well, this carried on for a few weeks. One Thursday morning I woke up and I decided I had enough. I called him and asked for him to meet me at my home that morning. I told him, "If you are not *on* my way, then you are *in* my way." I continued, I have to release you from this leadership position and we can no longer work on this together because I am no longer going to be held back. I have to remove all the obstacles in my way. I took this position not because I was looking for a position. I took it not for the position but because I had a vision.

Never take a position in life. Take a vision. This is why people 70% of people dislike their jobs and their position. You want vision, not position. Whenever one takes a job for a position, it is only a matter of time where they will be very unhappy. Normally within the first 9 months of that position, they will be looking outside again. I had to let that person go. Do I like letting people go? No. I have had to fire hundreds of people in my life. Is it ever nice? No. Is there ever a nice way of doing it? Not really. I lost a friendship for about 8 years, though we did reunite again.

When breaking a habit, you have to be looking at a new trajectory. Your friends and others you associate with are a vital component. I want to tell you that 95% of your success or failure in breaking habits has to do with the people you associate yourself with and hang out with.

How important is your breaking the habit to you? Is it everything? Is it just a little thing in your life? If you have habits that you want to break, you are going to have to re-evaluate the people in your life. How hungry are you for you being successful in breaking your habit that is holding you back? Just a little? Are you prepared to give up some friends, family and even some associates? Ouch. "Oh no Kurt, please don't ask me to do that?" Yip, I am asking you to do that. You may have to change the company you have been working with.

Put on your safety belts now, some of you are about to get really upset with me. I am about to offend some people. I do not want to offend anyone, but if you choose to get offended, please give me some grace. Here it is, hold on tight. In extreme cases, you may have to get a divorce. What? Some may have to. I am not telling you to get a divorce, or saying that if your spouse is holding you back get a new one, trade him or her in. What I will tell you is, there are some extreme cases where that may have to happen. I will never forget when a woman told me she wanted to divorce her husband. I said no, don't. I said work through it. She said that she could no longer work through it. I said, you have just about been married for 20 years, you can make this happen. She said no. About 6 months after that she filed for divorce. I was not happy as I know them both really well. A few years later I was chatting to her and found out what was happening behind the closed front door. I was shocked. I could not believe what I was hearing. I had no idea that was happening in their marriage. Even when I asked her at the time when she originally told me, what is happening that you want you divorce him? She only told me a few things. She was protecting him even though she wanted to divorce him. I made a decision that I will never again tell someone not to get divorced as we don't totally know what happens behind closed front doors. The right thing was for her to divorce that person because her life turned upside down. Her life changed radically. She started doing triathlons, running, making many new friends, started excelling in her career and so much confidence came to her that she could take on anything. The best thing she ever did was to get divorced. Yes, uncles and aunts did not support her and even her kids held it against her as did some friends. Years later, her kids said,

"Mom, I now totally understand why you divorced Dad."

You will need to divorce or separate some people, projects, associations in your life in order to break some habits. Some will need to divorce and some you will limit your association with. So many people keep living with habits they need to break because they have a fear of limiting some associations. So many people will not give up associations and friends and therefore will never ever break certain habits. This is a vitally important part of breaking bad habits, actually, 95% of you breaking your "Big Bad Habit" has to do with the people you are hanging out with.

Mistake #5: Isolation with No Accountability

Research shows that people who have accountability in their lives, generally live healthier lives. That accountability may come from family or friends. Research also shows that organizations that have accountability, perform at higher levels with greater profits and have happier employees. Countries that have governments with checks and balances systems between their executive, legislative and judicial divisions have healthier and transparent operations. Of course, there is no perfect system or people yet the level of operation is far higher when there are greater levels of accountability. No matter the operation, size or unit, accountability with transparency always wins. We have seen and watched dictatorships around the world come and go, from Africa, Central and South America, Eastern Europe, Cuba and the rest of the world. Where there is limited accountability, there is limited productivity. For many reasons people tend to isolate themselves when it comes to breaking habits and accountability. Those successful at breaking bad habits all have had some form of accountability. People think they can go alone or do it alone when breaking bad habits.

There is less effort when people are holding one accountable when breaking habits. Why? Well, with accountability comes a certain amount of internal guilt and personal internal disappointment. One does not want to let someone else down. Also, the majority of human beings tend to want to please others, especially ones that they have a relationship with.

Avoid isolation. Isolation is one of the most arrogant, prideful attitudes you get on this planet. The thought that you don't need anyone or anything to help you is ludicrous. We are created beings with dependencies. Just the fact that one battles to break a bad habit, shows that one is already dependent on something, the habit.

I have a friend who claims to be very wealthy. I don't spend much time with him anymore because of his arrogance and attitude and that is exactly what I do not want to become. He claims how independent he is and how he does not need anyone in his life. At the same time, he continually searches for someone to meet certain needs of his. We all have needs and there are certain basic needs a human has that only other humans can meet. The arrogance of believing we can do this alone is ludicrous.

There are no self-made millionaires on this planet. Somewhere I will show you they got some help from someone. breaking your Big Bad Habit (BBH), is going to take some help. Isolation is defeat. Countries that are isolated are defeated. Look at South Africa and all its false pride with its white racial "Apartheid" regime. That system led to is isolation and eventual downfall.

The Comprehensive Anti-Apartheid Act of 1986 was passed by the US Congress, first by the House of Representatives and then the Senate. It was then vetoed by President Reagan and then the President's veto was overridden. This presidential override by Congress was marked as the first time in the twentieth century that a president had a foreign policy veto overridden.

This act of Congress led to a massive isolation. There were 23 prohibitions and many other policies and procedures that isolated South Africa. Prohibitions such as the following:

- Importation of krugerrands
- Importation of military articles
- Importation of products from parastatal organizations
- Computer exports to South Africa
- Loans to the Government of South Africa
- Air transportation with South Africa (which meant no more PanAM to South Africa)
- Nuclear trade with South Africa

- Government of South Africa bank accounts
- Importation of uranium and coal from South Africa
- New investment in South Africa
- Promotion of United States tourism in South Africa (which never actually occurred)
- Importation of iron and steel
- Exports of crude oil and petroleum products
- Cooperation with the armed forces of South Africa (which did not totally happen as the USA supported South African Defense Force in fighting Cubans flying Russian Migs over Angola in 1987 and 1988)
- Sugar imports.

There were many embargoes, laws and resolutions passed by many countries, the United Nations and many organizations such as the Olympic Games expelling and denying South Africans from any games as early as 1970.

Embargos were passed and other rulings such as South African Airways was banned and denied the rights to fly over many African countries and therefore the airline had to fly around the bulge of

Africa to Europe. South African Airways was not allowed to fly to the USA in 1986, and then in 1987, it was denied to fly to Australia.

Disinvestment campaigns and the laws passed in the USA isolated the country economically, culturally, militarily, and financially. The disinvestment from major corporations devalued the South African Rand (currency) and inflation rose between 12 and 15% per year. South Africa was forced to change its policies and laws.

If there is anyone who understands isolation, it is a South African. I first visited the USA in March 1990, which was a month after Nelson Mandela had been released from his 27-year prison sentence. I stayed in youth hostels all across the USA. I met young people across the USA at the youth hostels. Every single day, there were people at all the hostels from all over the world and I had questions being fired at me about South Africa. Only a few were contentious, yet the feeling of isolation was all over. It seemed there was the world, and then there was South Africa. Every question seems to have had some attachment to the isolation of my birth country.

Neither countries nor individuals are liberated by isolation. Prisoners of War, such as John McCain, never experienced freedom in isolation. He felt confident and stronger away from isolation because as humans we were created to work in teams, in groups, in families and with other people. We were not created to be separated for long periods of time.

We were not designed to fight our battles by ourselves. We need others to win the battles and wars.

Unfortunately, when people go through a rough time they tend to do either of 2 things. They either bury their head in the sand and isolate themselves or they cannot keep their mouth quiet and they tell the whole world. We need each other, and we need to be accountable. We all need it.

Mistake #6: Environments Not Conducive to Change

The Wright brothers knew that the conditions needed to be right when attempting their first flight. They had to make sure which environment would have the right conditions. They needed wind for lift. When forming habits, you may have to change your environment so that the conditions are optimal. If you are creating a habit to support your healthy lifestyle, then perhaps it would be good to change your environment of hanging out at the local hamburger joint or the local neighborhood tavern. If you are creating a habit free from smoke, then change your environment and don't eat at restaurants that have an outside smoking section. This sounds like common sense. Well, common sense ain't so common when forming habits.

Environment just makes things easier, look better and feel better when forming habits. I love playing with words. Why? Well, I am dyslexic. I cannot see certain things in words and sentences or sometimes I see things that aren't even there in a word or sentence. Forming a habit or breaking habits where the environment is not supporting the habit will not help you break a habit. You may have to change your environment. You may have to change your friends or place where you hang out.

"Chains of habit are too light to be felt until they are too heavy to be broken."
– Warren Buffett

Chapter 3: The Bridge

A broken bad habit should always be replaced by a GREAT HABIT!

If you remove something without replacing something, you create a void or sometimes a vacuum. This is a universal rule or even a universal law. When we create a vacuum or void, often this leads to chaos. We saw this when the USA went into Iraq. There was no real exit strategy. The vacuum and void led to chaos.

The first time a father or mother leaves his/her family to go away for an extended period of time, there seems to be a vacuum. My father often travels for business. They were generally short trips from being away from his family. I will never forget in July 1979 when my dad left South Africa for his first overseas trip. He was flying literally around the world and was only coming back in September. I will never forget us standing at the airport in Johannesburg and watching the Boeing 747 take off. We watched it until we could not see it. I remember the tears my mom had in her eyes. No one in our extended family had really done what my dad was doing. Our family seemed to be in a vacuum. My mother held it together and did what she could to keep the family normal without my dad.

I will never forget when my mother went away for a week. This was the first time since I was born. I must have been around 10 or 11 years old. The family was in a vacuum and in chaos for a week. That was the biggest void I have ever experienced. Fathers can go away, but mothers, ahhhh I don't know about that. I have a friend whose mother and father walked out, and the kids were left to themselves. I know the chaos that they went through. Yet, he has turned out a phenomenal business owner and father and husband.

Breaking a habit that has controlled your life for a long time requires a big replacement of another habit or a few smaller habits. Many small "behaviors" or little actions will be needed to fill the void. Without filling the so-called void with smaller habits or actions, the tendency for the old habit will come back far more easily. Less discipline and willpower will be needed to break the old habit if one has begun to form a new habit. Modern science has proved that forming good habits decreases other bad behaviors and invigorates other good behaviors. Also, the more good habits that are formed, the fewer amounts of discipline and willpower are necessary to create other good habits.

Immediately forming a new habit and actions that are repetitive is vital. This is the reason why many have battled to pack the old habit up. This is why New Year's resolutions do not work 91% of the time.

It is so much easier breaking a bad habit when you are focusing on a new habit. If you want to reduce the amount of discipline and the amount of willpower when breaking a habit, simply replace the old bad habit with a new habit. You may have to start a few small new good habits to replace the one Big Bad Habit. Limiting your need for willpower to break the old habit is having the will to say *No* and the power to say *Yes* to the new habit. The more Yeses you say to the new habit, the easier it is for you say No to the old habit.

I have witnessed hundreds of people who have not managed to give up smoking cigarettes. I smoked for quite some years. I know the hell that I went through to pack it up. I tried giving it up and struggled for a long time. I learnt that to give this habit up, I needed to avoid the 5 mistakes mentioned above, but also had to create new and exciting habits that would re-direct my mind, thoughts and images away from wanting it. I had to find other things to do. It was about action and meaning. Smoking or other bad habits are normally filling a void in one's life. The reason why one starts bad habits in the first place, is one is filling a need. Someone said to me, "I started smoking not because of a need, but I wanted to stay cool with my friends (when it was still cool to smoke)." I said yes, and that was a need you were meeting. You had a need to be accepted by your peers. Your behavior was meeting a need. You were insecure without your friends' acceptance. We all seem to have a need to be accepted in our lives at some point. Some have that need throughout life. Others seem to only have that need from their inner circle, family or their closest friends.

Breaking a "Big Bad Habit" should only be decided upon when a new habit or repetitive set of actions and behaviors have been decided upon.

"Once you learn to quit, it becomes a habit."

– Vince Lombardi

Chapter 4: Who Decides the Future?

Breaking bad habits is not just about breaking something negative: cigarettes, alcohol, drugs, overeating or anything you are putting into your body in excess. Breaking habits can be breaking a habit that is not necessarily bad for you but a habit that is limiting you from reaching a dream, vision, goal, campaign or purpose. You may have a plan to complete a triathlon. In order for you to do this, you need to train in the mornings before going off to work. You have had a habit of reading the newspaper or getting online and reading the breaking news every day while sipping your coffee. Reading and catching up on local events can help you in communicating better with people and connecting with others. It is not necessarily a bad habit, but a habit that is not getting you where you want to get to.

The first step is deciding what you want to become. You may say, in 6 months I want to complete a triathlon, or run a 5K, or get a promotion in my company or have a vacation in Europe. The question is, what habits will you need to break that will hold you back from achieving your goal. Normally when we want to go to another level, we need to grow into something. Things don't just happen. We normally need to grow into what we want to become.

Getting hungry to grow opens new doors of thought that will make you want to break some habits and start some new ones. Like a little kid says to their parents, "Measure me, Mom, have I grown?" I remember wondering if I had grown. I would say "Let me see how I have grown" ... It is natural for us to want to grow. So sad how adults grow up and then lose the desire to grow. They lose the desire to grow in knowledge, grow emotionally, relationally and spiritually. Adults seem to grow when they try new clothes on, they realize they have grown. All they were to do is grow smaller, just like their mental, emotional and knowledge growth. Little kids, all they want is to grow. We have a desire to grow. I have never heard a kid burst out crying and say "Oh no, Mom, I have grown again, please can I stop growing?" They may cry because they did not grow. As a kid I used to have terrible cramps in my legs. My mom always told me that it was growing pains. One day as a kid I got to the fridge to take milk out the fridge and I could reach the milk and I said "Mom, Mom, I have grown." The growing pains really work … I can reach the milk … The thing I did not know was that my mom had cleaned the fridge and changed the height of the fridge shelf. I thought I had grown. It was about perception.

> *If people don't decide their futures, then who does?*

Growing into the person we want to become is going to cause us growing pains. The things that hold us back in our life are bad habits. Habits either take us to our successes and dreams, or they imprison us. The process of breaking habits can be painful. There are growing pains in breaking habits and creating new ones. As a kid we were taught how to handle growing pains. When we get older we just seem to hunger for comfort and sprint away from pain, forgetting this life is a marathon, not a sprint.

Perhaps the question should be, "if people don't decide their futures, then *what* decides your future?" I have always loved this quote:

"People do not decide their futures, they decide their habits and their habits decide their futures."
— F. M. Alexander.

We ask children what do you want to become when you are older? We ask adults the same question but in a different way. We always focus on the "What." What do you want to become, or what do you want to do with your life? Very few questions are ever asked, on "**what**" will you do to achieve that. People who succeed are the ones who focus on "what" they will do to achieve success. People who take their lives from being successful to the top 5% who operate at a high level of success are the ones who don't just focus on *what* they are going to do but *how* they are going to do it.

The "How" question will either make you or break you.

So many people when starting a project, goal or dream, if they first ask "How," they can be easily paralyzed just by the thought of it. Thinking about the "How" will they achieve that can cause them not to even start because of the fear of doing it. Although the how is critical to succeed at a higher level, the same how can cripple and paralyze one.

My advice to anyone starting a business or a training program or just about any goal, is not to be overwhelmed by the "How." Someone else has probably done it before. Start with the "what" and get coached by an expert on the "How."

Too many people stop working toward the big future because they got intimidated by the big "How." The big "How" will make you or break you. When your goal takes momentum, start focusing on the "How."

Where can I learn the "How"? Coaching is number one. You get what you pay for, right. Hire a cheap, inexpensive coach and that is what you may end up with. Hire a coach that is dynamic and may cost more, you will probably get the best advice that will also cause you to succeed at a higher level.

Do research on getting the right coach before choosing one. It took me 6 years to find the right speaking coach. It was not overnight when I found the right coach. I was looking for someone who could break some of the barriers and limitations in me.

I found this coach when I least expected to. In fact, the first few minutes of seeing him present at a conference I was not impressed. Ten minutes into his speech, I realized this is the coach for which I had been looking for 6 years. He told a story that impacted me. It was his story that I could identify with. The average person tends to identify more with people's failures than their successes.

When we meet someone who is earning millions of dollars per year, we may not truly be able to identify with them. We may say, "Wow, I would like to earn that or achieve that or do what they are doing," but still do not truly identify with them. So when this coach started talking about his failures, I immediately identified with him. He started to tell us habits that he had to break and overcome to get where he wanted to be. Because of his failure, that I could identify with and watch him go from zero to 3 million dollars per year, I could easily relate to him. I needed the "How" and not just the "What." The whole process of "Identification" is a powerful process of us achieving what we want to.

Although building a habit serves us in effectively breaking a bad habit, we use habits to build the life we desire. Habits are the foundation and often the cornerstone of us achieving our dreams. Forming a new habit is far more than just replacing a new habit for a bad habit, but is to build an exciting future and a dream.

Identify

How the heck do I identify what habits I should first break and which habits I will form? The foundation of your decision should be based on the end goal. What do you want to become? What do you want your legacy to be? What do you want to achieve or be known as? When you know what you want to become and who you want to become, then you need to identify the habits you need to break that are holding you back from achieving your dream and the great habits you need to form so that you can become that person.

A coach or a mentor will help you to identify this. Going to the next level will require you to form new habits and end old habits. Not all old habits are bad, they just no longer fulfill a purpose. A new trajectory demands new habits. A new trajectory requires breaking and ending old habits that have lost value in terms of what you would like to accomplish. The difference between successful people and high level top 5% of successful people is the habits that separate them. Your daily routine (habit driven) is the foundation of your success. All top performers in any field have mastered their habits.

You do not decide your future. It is your habits that decide your future. It is all about the habit.

Decision

Decisions are the place where habits are born. There is nothing like a powerful decision, a dedicated decision. Most success is birthed at decision and is a result of decision. What drives us to decision? The 2 factors that lead us to decision making are emotions and logic. We make decisions based on logic, but we act on emotion. When there is a movement of emotion in us, and we add logic to it, a decision is made. When we take action based on that dedicated decision, and we repeat the action over time, we get a habit.

David Romero, CEO of CENTURY 21 AWARD, a mentor and a boss of mine for over 15 years who has remained a mentor, taught me about the meaning of the "ci" in the word *decision*. I will never forget that lesson. In the word de$\underline{ci}$sion we see the letters "ci." There are 4,000 words in the English language associated with or have the "ci" in it. Where ever you see the "ci," the word will be related to either separating, cutting off, destroying or even killing. Take words such as *herbicide* (a toxic substance that is used to destroy unwanted vegetation), *pesticide* (a substance used for destroying insects that are harmful to plants or to animals), *circumscribe* (to draw a line around, therefore separating), *vaccination* (inoculation with a vaccine in order to protect against a particular disease therefore cutting off a potential disease), *incision* (a surgical cut made in skin or flesh),

homicide (the deliberate killing of one person by another; murder) **genocide** (the deliberate killing of massive amounts of people, especially those of a particular ethnic group or nation), *circumcise* (to remove or cut off the foreskin of a male's penis) *suicide* (the act of killing oneself) and another 3,993-plus words.

The word De*ci*sion also has the "ci" in it. Every time we make a decision, we are either separating, cutting off, destroying or even killing something. The average human makes on average 15,000 to 30,000 decisions per day. We are actually separating something, cutting off something or someone, destroying something or someone or even killing something or someone. Every time I decide to take a sip of water, I am killing thirst. All of us are a bunch of murderers. We make on average 2,500 decisions per day on eating and drinking.

We are killing things all the time. We all kill the spirit of other people. We take away their humor, their self-confidence and their self-belief without even realizing it. We do it to ourselves as well, in fact we do it more often than not. We have killed our dreams, visions and greatness in our life. We have cut off our great futures and separated our futures that potentially we have. We do this all the time.

70% of our decisions come from our non-conscious. We make decisions based on our non-conscious all the time and we are not even conscious of it. Have you ever walked into a grocery store and purchased something and then got home and thought why did I buy that? I did not even go to the store for that. Have you ever bought a big-ticket item and even a day later thought, why on earth did I ever buy that? We do that because of seeds and thoughts that have been put into our mind and stored away in our non-conscious. This happens through watching television, listening to a radio ad, listening to podcasts, documentaries, reading, magazines, Facebook and social media posts, talking to friends, and even being at a Starbucks coffee shop and your non-conscious hearing someone saying something at another table. Our non-conscious is extremely powerful and controls much of our life.

Having a dream, vision, cause, campaign, mission or a planned destiny without a strategy to break bad habits and create great habits is like hoping to win the lottery without buying a ticket. No matter how much you hope and wish to win the lottery, it will never happen without buying a ticket. I have never heard of anyone winning the lottery without buying a ticket. Having a dream, vision, cause, campaign, mission or a planned destiny without a strategy to break bad habits and create great habits is like a pilot getting on a commercial airline and taking off and not having any GPS coordinates, no navigation system and not pressurizing the cabin. It just ain't going to get there.

I was watching CNN reporting about the so-called terrible hurricane "Florence" in September 2018 about to hit the Carolinas. I have some close friends who live in Jacksonville, North Carolina and I was concerned as they had not evacuated. The weather reporters were pretty accurate on how the storm was about to hit. I remember how Anderson Cooper, Don Lemon and Chris Cuomo repeatedly said, "Do not run a generator in your house or even in your garage." I heard the Weather Channel say exactly the same thing so many times again and again. In fact, I got tired of hearing it. I thought, come on, guys, we get it. The storm had not even gone through yet; they were reporting that a couple in their early 60s had passed away from carbon monoxide poisoning in South Carolina because they had their generator running in their home. I also realized that many had lost power so they did not see that or hear that. Then I thought, well, if they had a generator then they would have potentially had the opportunity to hear them say that on their television, radio or internet. Decisions we make can seem good, but actually kill us without us even knowing it. With all the technology, all the power (even from a personal generator) we can live in a bubble and not do the right things to save ourselves or protect ourselves. This leads us into the next chapters.

"People do not decide their futures, they decide their habits and their habits decide their futures."

– F. M. Alexander

Chapter 5: Habit Forming

I have learned and seen in my own life and others', that people often know *what* to do, but not *how*. Many CEOs, COOs, Regional Managers, sales professionals, and many other careers know what to do, but have not researched, studied, asked or learnt the "How to do it."

Knowing is the enemy of learning. I want to say that again. *Knowing is the enemy of learning.* This is one of the most frightening, realistic and truthful thoughts. I have watched people in different industries who have been around a long time and they say, "Been there, done that, bought the T-shirt."

When one believes that they know something, the tendency is to move into something else and to keep on teaching what you have already learnt. The danger of that is being left behind.

We have watched companies go out of business because they assumed that their enemy was their competition. Companies like Blockbuster, Borders and hundreds of others. These names are a cliché now when talking about companies not moving fast enough.

Your enemy is not your competition. Your biggest enemy is yourself. It is that you think you know it. Your knowledge is your biggest enemy to yourself, your career, your ability to develop, to research, to grow, to engage.

Every generation fights the upcoming generation's cultural changes. Just look at music. How many times have I heard a previous generation run down the new generation's music, clothes, hair styles and slang language?

Knowing what to do is not good enough anymore. Knowing _how_ to act, behave, connect, build and communicate with yourself and others is critical. Because habits are based on repetitive actions and behaviors, your actions and behaviors are critical in forming habits that are relevant and connect with the new social culture and business culture. I have watched businesses and business professionals act in ways that are so irrelevant in terms of the direction the culture is changing. If you have children, ask yourself, "How are my children relating to me and my behaviors?"

Many people think they are stuck. Stuck in a career, job, city, state, rut, box, circumstance, way of doing something, or environment. People are not really stuck. All they are is actually committed to certain patterns of behaviors because they actually worked for them in the past. Those behaviors did work in the past, but no longer serve the same purpose. So often, people cannot progress because they keep on applying old formulas and habits. Change the habit, formula, structure and behavior and you will be shocked at your results.

Decide on actions and behaviors that will form habits that will not only help you break bad habits, but will serve your dreams, goals, campaigns and your family.

"Procrastination is the bad habit of putting off until the day after tomorrow what should have been done the day before yesterday." **– Napoleon Hill**

Chapter 6: HABIT

All of us are creatures of habit. We form habits quicker than we are too often willing to admit.

Here are five simple ways to form Great Healthy Habits.

Let's look at the word HABIT.

H - Humble

Take a humble approach to creating a Big Great Habit. Too many start too big or with too many habits and then nothing materializes. Being humble means to plan in small steps. I will never forget the night before I was about to do my first international Ironman triathlon. I had just immigrated 7 months before to the USA and was living in Phoenix, Arizona. I was training in the heat day after day. The ironman triathlon includes a swim of 3.8 km (2.4 miles), 180 km (112 miles) and then a full marathon of 42 km (26 miles). The night before the race, my father, who is and was an Ironman legend (still, I believe, the oldest African to complete an Ironman at 78 years old), called me from South Africa. My dad called me to wish me the best of luck for the next day. My dad had completed many Ironman Triathlons and shorter triathlons so he had earned the right to advise me. He gave me two pieces of advice. I will share one of them now. He said "Kurt, if you want to finish this race, you need to humble yourself or this race will humble you." I have learnt that when trying to achieve something big and to have a breakthrough, one needs to humble yourself or it will humble you. Taking on a big habit will humble you if you do not humble yourself. When taking on something big, start small. You cannot go from not working out to working out 2 hours. You cannot go from not training on a bicycle to riding 180 km. Even an an Ironman, I would advise an inspired athlete to first attempt a sprint distance or an Olympic distance or even a half Ironman before attempting the full Ironman.

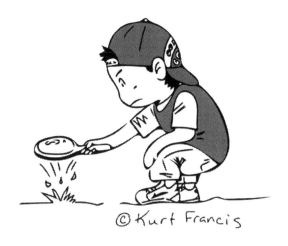

© Kurt Francis

If you start forming a big habit, even when replacing a bad habit, have a clear focus on what you are doing. We all know that if we take a magnifying glass and we keep it focused on a piece of paper without moving it, it starts smoldering and eventually the paper catches on fire. This is one of the greatest lessons we learn as a kid. However, we forget this lesson really fast. Our lives have things thrown at us every single minute. Information is flying at us all the time and we have so many interruptions with notifications literally screaming at us all the time. When you are building a habit, you need to keep your eyes, mind, direction and focus on one thing, the habit. If we took this magnifying glass and moved it around all the time, we would not achieve the result we wanted or expected.

Setting ambitious and big goals is great, but starting big with massive steps is not always smart. In fact, I highly recommend starting with small little steps. I mean smaller than you think. This applies to giving up bad habits as well. Just as if you decide to quit putting sugar in your body, and you suddenly stop, your endeavors could end within your first 30 days and you could be back on sugar and eating double the amount. This is one of the major causes of failure of habit forming. This is why many fail at New Year's resolutions.

While you might initially feel inspired and energized by setting a big and massive "blowout" and life transforming habits for your New Year, your inspiration and energy can fade away at lightning speed. Resolutions can be made really quickly, but the physical urges come back really fast. There is nothing wrong with making a decision with forming a massive ginormous habit. That is not the problem. The problem is starting off with the big habit. This is the number one reason why people fail.

Small, incremental lifestyle changes may feel and look less attractive, but they will have a much greater chance of creating real life long changes. According to Dr. Roberta Anding, a registered dietician and nutrition professor at Baylor College of Medicine, moderating your resolutions could be the difference between giving up in February and creating a lasting lifestyle change.

When our Big Great Habit goals are too ambitious, we struggle to change our habits. We become discouraged quickly, tend to fail fast and ultimately give up. The danger of this is not just giving up, but sowing a seed in your mind that you are a failure when creating habits. In the future you will already have a negative thought about forming habits. You must start training your brain again. So instead of making another resolution, start humbly using the My Epoch Challenge for forming lifelong habits. What is My Epoch Challenge? I am so glad you asked. I will give more details about it later.

H - Habit

A - Accountability

Accountability is something humans tend to hate. At the same time, when they don't get it, they blame the company, organization or their boss for not getting it. What I have experienced in managing thousands of people, no matter who the person is, everyone wants a leader even when they deny wanting one or needing one. Even the biggest thug or gang member wants a leader, a gang leader. Dictators even want leaders. They want information or some resource that will lead them. Everyone is looking for something. Accountability is much the same way. People often hate it when they are held accountable but desire the praise, recognition and the rewards it offers. I have worked closely with salespeople, some of them earning in excess of $1 million per year. Whether earning $100,000 per year or a million dollars per year, people want recognition. You don't get recognition without accountability.

There are very few things in life that come without accountability. To be rich, you need accountability. To serve, you need accountability. The best producers, achievers and performers want and desire accountability, especially when they are doing well. The best producers, achievers and performers want coaches. Good coaches take people to the next level.

Anyone who is serious about forming a habit to get them to the next level, no matter what that level is, needs to have accountability. Accountability can come in a form of a coach, a spouse, a business partner, a co-worker, a friend, a relative, or even a neighbor.

Accountability requires important criteria to be effective. #1. Very clear expectations on the results by a given time. #2. Very clear expectations on the actions or activities that need to be achieved by a given time, weekly or monthly. #3. Regular communication between the two parties. #4. The format of the weekly/monthly communication must be agreed on. Will it be in person, a video/visual format (such as FaceTime, Skype, Zoom, text or email. I highly recommend video or visual formats because parties cannot multitask while meeting and body language and facial expressions reveal a lot. This accountability may even be done in a group format with many others. Group accountability has greater effect as people are often more concerned with what their peers think of them than the leader or coach.

True authentic accountability is when you have risen to the level of holding yourself accountable at a high level and using systems such as My Epoch Challenge does. When one reaches the level of self-accountability, and succeeds at that, one is ready to move on to mastery. This is another whole discussion on its own. Self-accountability in conjunction with others holding you accountable is a giant step toward achieving success in forming a great habit that can change and "transvigorate™" your life.

H - Humble

A - Accountability

B - Believe

A few years ago, I had a memorable experience attending a basketball game at San Diego State University (SDSU). An acquaintance of mine had complained to me about not being able to get tickets. Luckily for me, I had a connection that was able to hook me up. I'll never forget the excitement I felt over being able to attend that sold out game!

A friend told me a story about he and his son heading down to the same game. While in route, his son told him "Dad, drive faster, I don't want to be late." The father said, "the game starts at 4 pm and it is 3 pm now." His son replied, "Dad, it is not about the game, it is about the show." I learnt and experienced that the show starts 30 minutes before the game starts.

Wow, believe me, the show starts a half hour before. I have never ever been to such an exciting game (show) before in my life. The whole deal is a performance, from the music to the Aztec mascot. Everyone is involved. The crowd goes crazy even before the game begins. They have an incredible chant called "I Believe." The whole stadium erupts and gets involved. It is impossible to sit there and not be caught up by all the emotion, energy and enthusiasm.

The chant goes like this, "I believe, I believe that, I believe that we, I believe that we will, I believe that we will win."

This sounds just like words. Oh no it is not. With music and all the energy, it feels like you are at a concert.

This team went from being around 200th in position in the rankings to making the sweet 16. March Madness became a mad time for any San Diegan.

How does a team go from 200 to the top 16? It is impossible not to believe when you are in an environment of 30,000 people going crazy. When your environment has this supernaturally inspired and invigorated belief, you cannot but win. It is hard to lose in an environment like that.

The belief mental state was changed not just by the team, but by all the spectators, fans and just everyone. It was not about the game; it was about the show.

This SDSU basketball team had a phenomenal coach, Coach Steve Fisher. To take a team from 200th position to the sweet 16 is something. I love his humility. When asked about the success of the team and his success as a coach, this is what Coach Fisher replied, "It's not me, it's we …"

When we are 21 years old, we believe we can do anything. When we reach 40 years old and the world has slapped us sideways, we don't believe in anything.

Well, let me stop there. That is not my belief. I have some school friends who are just existing and all they do is watch TV, complain about politics and talk about their retirement. Retirement is for people who don't have a campaign in life. So many lose hope and belief. So many give up on their life and their friends' lives. I see so many people encouraging others not to do something or not to take a risk.

How do we restore our belief when we get to 40 or 50 years old? How do we get back to when we were 21 years old and believed that we could do anything we put our minds to?

I learnt from Muhammad Ali something that impacted my life. I have taken what he said and expanded it a little bit. I will never forget how I felt when I heard this. He said, "It is the repetition of affirmations that lead to belief. And once this belief becomes a deep conviction, things begin to happen." I have changed this a little for my life. I say, "It is the relentless repetition and rehearsals of self-affirmations that leads, restores and revives my belief. When this belief becomes a deep conviction, something begins to happen and manifest in my life." People say, "Well I don't believe that I can do that anymore. I am too old, Kurt." They are 100% correct. Another person who is 20 years older can say, "I believe I can do that" and they are correct. It is about belief. If you are struggling with your belief, you can break through in a powerful way.

Write down some powerful affirmations. Write them down as if you are achieving them now. Put them on your mobile device. Read them aloud in the morning, again at 10 am, again at lunch time, again at 3 pm, again at 6 pm and again before going to bed. Stand up if you can, say them out loud. Pretend you are doing a rehearsal in front of 5,000 people. Visualize that you are on stage, thousands are watching you. Feel the experience. You may think this is crazy. Are you looking to break through? Are you hungry enough? Are you willing to fight for what is there waiting for you or are you going to just give up and lie on the couch watching *Judge Judy*? Proclaim that this is what is happening in your life. I am telling you, that you will be shocked at what happens. When you keep on repeating and rehearsing your affirmation, it will become a deep conviction and when this deep conviction happens, then something will manifest and begin to happen. I ask people what is happening their life. They say "nothing" or "same old thing ..." If nothing is happening in your life it means that there is no conviction. If there is no conviction it means you are not fighting for something. When you get in a room, close the door and start doing your affirmations. So, do you want something to happen in your life or not? If not, then get on the couch. If you want to form some new habits, and to take back your life and control your future, start with affirmations. Your belief will rise, you will get convicted and something powerful will happen and manifest itself.

Earlier in Chapter One, we discussed how, if we want to break a habit, we need to stop talking about it.

Every time you talk about your undesirable bad habit, pinch yourself. I learnt this lesson when living in Charlotte, North Carolina. I was driving routes for FedEx Ground. I was doing an average of 80 stops per day and driving between 200 and 300 miles per day. I was working between 12 and 14 hours per day. My longest day was 19 hours, just before Christmas. I was going through a rough time in my life. Although I was achieving well while at FedEx, I started hating my life. I had terrible thoughts go through my mind. I will never forget how I had to fight those thoughts. I remember us experiencing a terrible storm in 2002/2003 in Charlotte, North Carolina. It was freezing rain. There was no electricity for 5 days and the city had just about closed down. My apartment had no electricity. No hot water to shower and working 14 hours plus per day. I did not even want to go home to an empty, cold, dark apartment. My emotions were low and seemed like they were getting lower. I kept on having these terrible thoughts. Thoughts that I did not want to live anymore. These thoughts became more regular. Eventually, these thoughts filled my mind. I remember I came to a decision that something had to change. This was a Ground Zero for me. I was looking for an explosion point. I had hit rock bottom.

Many things were happening to me at that time. I had recently come out to my family and friends that I was gay. Although my family accepted me, and went out of their way for me, I knew that they did not understand. I did not expect them to. I learned that many deleted me and broke relationships with me. My life needed a breakthrough. I learned that I had to change my behavior which had become a bad habit and stop talking like that even to myself.

Bad habits are not only our behavior. Bad habits start off with the conscious and then become non-conscious. 70% of our decisions are non-conscious. We train our brain to think in a certain way by repetition. Have you ever walked into a grocery store and purchased things and got back home and said to yourself, "Why did I buy that? That is not even the reason I went to the store." We make more decisions based on our non-conscious than our conscious. The dangerous habits are the ones we have taught our brain and when our non-conscious starts tapping into what we have trained it; it is very difficult to break that pattern or habit.

You will learn how I changed this when I talk about creating great habits.

I started using my tongue and saying things that I did not even feel. That is right, I started using my tongue and my mouth and started saying things that I totally did not feel. I started speaking success and breakthrough. I had to break the habit of bad thoughts. We tend to say what we feel like. We tend to speak what we feel like. Taking back your life when you don't feel like it is not easy but possible. Taking control of your life is not easy when your emotions are not where they need to be, but it is possible. Changing your direction is not easy but is possible. Our feelings will lie to us. Our feelings will not always tell us the truth. Our feelings will not always tell us our destiny, our purpose, our dream, our vision nor our campaign. Breaking a bad, undesirable, unwanted habit is not always easy, but it can become easier when we understand the process and where our power lies. You were given a tongue and it was not only given to you to swallow, chew food like a lollipop or ice cream, or make sounds, or use the 10,000 taste buds to distinguish between bitter, salty, sweet or sour, protect you from poison and to manipulate food for digestion. Your tongue was given to you as a powerful muscle, a muscle that can redirect your life. Your tongue is used as a catalyst so that your brain can release neurochemicals. Your tongue is also not just a muscle but a survival mechanism. There is a connection between your tongue and brain, believe it or not! When speaking great things, your brain releases four chemicals: endorphins, oxytocin, serotonin and dopamine.

The way you talk about yourself, the words that come from your tongue about yourself, the words that come out of your mouth need to be controlled. The words that you speak out are training your brain. The words that your tongue speaks are training your non-conscious. You need to be saying about yourself what *your dream demands, your vision expects and your campaign desires.* Others are relying on what you say about yourself. People who have not learnt to discipline their tongues are the ones who live unfulfilled lives. These same people are the ones who are stuck in depression, poverty, always living in scarcity and the land of never enough, always believing bad things will happen to them, always believing that Murphy's Law is a natural law. They say things like, I can never do anything right, and that is why everything is never right. They say things like I am always late, and they are always late. They say "Nothing ever works out for me," and nothing ever does work out for them. I never have enough money, and they never do. They say that nobody wants to hang out with them and nobody does. They believe that everyone rejects them and everyone does reject them. Cut it out. *You will never go beyond your confession. Life will only give you what you speak out about. Life will only give you what you ask for, seek for. Your tongue controls your confession. When you confess it, that is it.*

Fight for your life. Stop sitting back and waiting for your life. Get out of bed, get out of that chair, close your door, start fighting for your life. Claim back and confess what is yours.

Your spirit is waiting for you.
Your mental state is waiting for you to do this.
Your physical body is waiting for you to do this.

Your dreams are waiting for this.

Your wealth, income, and career are waiting for this.

Your personal life is waiting for this.

Your relationships and family are waiting for this.

Your spouse is waiting for this.

Your kids are waiting for this.

Your co-workers are waiting for this.

Life is a battle and a fight for position. You are in a battle. Do warfare with your tongue. What others say to you may be important, but what you say to yourself is vitally important. What are you saying to yourself? Stop saying things that are not in alignment with your purpose. Start aligning your words with your destination. You were created for big things. Start saying big things over and over again. Stop saying bad things about others, they will come back to eat you. What comes out of your mouth reveals what is in your heart and your non-conscious. Listen to the words that come out of your mouth: humility or arrogance, fear or faith, greed or giving, jealousy or love for someone. Take your life back, take your authority back and speak out. Stop destroying your life with your words and then wondering why you cannot break through.

Your tongue is like a ship on the ocean. Your little tongue is a massive muscle, just like an aircraft … a large 747's direction is controlled by a small rudder. That small rudder redirects that aircraft. Let your rudder, your tongue start taking over. Take some affirmations and change your life. Start saying your home has favor. Your bank balance has favor. Your business has favor. Everything you do has favor. Your work has favor. Your family has favor. Let the world get a revelation that your whole life has favor. You have the authority to have favor on your life. You can have it right now. You don't have to wait. Your confession right now can turn everything around. You are going to have to make confession wonderful. Most people think confession is going to the priest and confessing. There is space for that, but the problem is they never move out of that habit, they create a habit of confessing wrongdoings and that is all. There is a confession of great things. Break out of the habit of only confessing wrongs, and start confessing things that this life wants to give you.

We have to rise above and let the power of our confession break through.

Nelson Mandela has been a massive inspiration to me. He said, "There is no passion to be found playing small - in settling for a life that is less than the one you are capable of living." If your life is playing small, it is time for you to start forming habits. Your life is not about you. The skills, gifts and talents you have are not for you; they are for you to help and serve others. If your life is small, then you are selfish and focused on your life. You may do small things, but those small things are big for others. People who live small lives are only pleasing themselves. When you live big, it means you are doing more for others than what you are doing for yourself. You may be a CEO of a massive company; you are living small if you are only doing for yourself. If you are a CEO, and you are doing it so that others in your company can achieve great things and that your clients can live better lives, then you are living big. Living big is not because of a position. A great position at a company is not about you but about how you can touch other people's lives. Live big. You may dislike Nelson Mandela. It does not matter if you do. He was given an opportunity to leave prison before he was released. He said, "No, don't release me, I am not in this prison because of me. I am in this prison because millions of people are counting on me to set them free."

We all believe in something. We believe we can or we believe we cannot. It is as simple as that. The power of belief will cause you to do something or not to do something. You want to live big and serve others, then form a habit. It is the habits in your life that decide your future.

H - Humble

A - Accountability

B - Believe

I - Indoctrination

Forming a habit is about teaching your life a set of behaviors, responses, actions and a new pattern of thinking. Indoctrination is a process of teaching yourself to accept a set of beliefs. You first need to have the belief, and now since you learnt to believe and how to restore your belief, it is time to accept the belief and apply it to your life in the form of behaviors and actions. When your belief becomes a deep conviction, and you start taking action based upon your deep conviction, you will see a habit start developing.

Habit forming is a process of teaching. The process is directly related to the repetition, not just repetition and rehearsal of words, but of actions as well. Becoming great at anything in life involves repetition and rehearsals. It is about doing something again and again.

Indoctrination when forming habits is the process of teaching yourself through repetitive action, behaviors and belief. It is about finding the deep conviction. Habits that are not related to a deep conviction, may not contribute to your life nor contribute to others around you at home or in your workplace.

Australian researchers Megan Oaten and Ken Cheng conducted a series of experiments focusing on the study of willpower being increased over time. They found a significantly large reduction in behaviors such as cigarettes smoked, alcohol consumed, junk food eaten, money spent impulsively, tempers flared, television watched, etc.

Developing different healthy habits over time invigorates other positive behaviors. When we indoctrinate our life with teaching great behaviors that leads into habits, we actually trick our body and life doing better things with less effort, less willpower and less discipline.

Creating one habit will lead you to create another good habit and will decrease other bad habits. Have you ever looked at very successful people and thought, wow they have so much discipline and so much willpower? You say to yourself, I wish I had so much discipline and willpower. Well, they don't have much more discipline and willpower than you. What they do have, is they have transformed their lives through forming habits. The initial habits cost them more willpower and more discipline. The more habits they created, the less willpower and discipline they needed to create other habits.

Forming great and powerful habits requires self-indoctrination. It starts within you.

H - Humble

A - Accountability

B - Believe

I - Indoctrination

T - Time

When we are young, time seems to take forever. As we get older, time seems to go so fast. We know that time heals many wounds and often pain. Things that are worth more tend to take longer to materialize or mature, from good wine even to cheese. We have learnt the saying my mother always taught us, "Easy come, easy go." The easier something comes, the easier something can go. The longer we work for something, the longer we will keep it. If we want good mature habits to stick around a long time in our life, it will take a little time to develop.

Extensive research has shown that forming a habit takes longer than 21 days, or 28 days. Different habits take different times to form. The sweet spot for a habit to form is 66 days, according to *The One Thing* by Gary Keller and Jay Papasan.

Forming a habit is very similar to an aircraft pilot's flight. Just like an aircraft, the pilots prepare for the flight. Once checks have occurred the aircraft heads for the runway and follows "taxiing" instructions to the correct runway. When the aircraft is cleared for takeoff, the pilot puts it on full throttle.

A flight by an aircraft has 5 or 6 phases. We will only discuss 3 of the phases that are relatable to building and forming a habit. The first phase is takeoff.

Phase One

As the pilot gives full throttle and power, the aircraft begins gaining speed. Although the aircraft gains tremendous speed it does not mean that it has enough speed to take off as there is not enough lift under the wings. Each aircraft has different speeds which are named specifically for aviation: V1, VR, VLOF and V2. These are termed as speeds, but they are actually related to the position of a runway.

V1 is the speed at which the "takeoff" should no longer be aborted because there is not enough runway left for the aircraft to stop safely. V1 position needs to be calculated before every takeoff, considering important facts such as the weight of the aircraft, the runway length, wing flap settings and aircraft brakes. Once an aircraft has reached V1 position, the pilot takes their hands off the throttle (power) and puts their hands on the rotator. The rotator is the yoke that lifts the aircraft off the ground.

The next speed is a VR or V Rotate which is the speed at which the pilot begins to apply control inputs to the aircraft's nose to pitch up where it will begin to leave the ground. This VR speed is also always calculated before takeoff. This is a point where the generated lift above the wings becomes higher than the weight of the aircraft and this is where the *front wheels* lift off the ground. Although the aircraft has lifted its front wheel off, the aircraft still has the back wheels touching the runway. The aircraft has started flying but has not taken off. Just like your habit, it has started flying but has not fully taken off yet. You are still using all your focus and willpower (full power from the engine) and discipline.

The next speed is VLOF which is the speed at which the aircraft *main wheels*, sometimes called the back wheels, lift off the ground. When the main wheels leave the ground, the aircraft has taken flight. Although one is flying, full power is still happening. Just like your habit, now is not the time to reduce your willpower or discipline.

Then there is V2, the speed which is called the "Takeoff Safety Speed," where if an aircraft had 2 engines, it could operate and maintain altitude with only 1 engine operating. This, pilots call "Obstacle Avoidance Procedures." Why do pilots consider this as a specific goal in their takeoff? Situations can occur during aircraft takeoff, such as an aircraft flying into birds, and only 1 engine then operates. We all know about the US Airways Flight 1549 landing on the Hudson River by Captain Sully on January 15th, 2009, as it hit birds and both engines went out. We may feel like we are flying, and the habit has taken flight, but we can still have obstacles that we will need to avoid.

As mentioned, research shows it takes 66 days for the average habit to form. Day 33 is when your habit starts to take flight. Although your habit has taken off, it is not yet formed until day 66. At day 99, we start cruising and we switch it on autopilot. Now the captain can use the *loo*! As we know, we may be at 33,000 feet, that does not mean no turbulence. Watch out! Check your radar and see if the weather ahead shows potential turbulence. Check your calendar and see if you may bump into

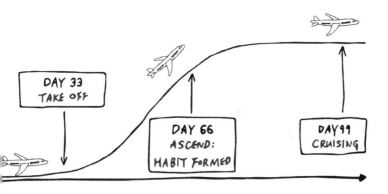

DAY 33
TAKE OFF

DAY 66
ASCEND:
HABIT FORMED

DAY 99
CRUISING

some people who may knock you off course with your habit.

Before you start forming your habit, you need to prepare. Just as pilots calculate their V1, VR, VLOF and V2 speeds or positions, we need to be ready and understand our habits taking off. It is a process and not an event. New habits start with a powerful decision. Tony Robbins calls it the moment of decision. Making decisions to start new habits without calculating like pilots do before takeoff, end up like most New Year's resolutions do, they just fizzle away or crash. At the moment of your decision when one commits oneself followed immediately by a plan and action, even the smallest action, the chance for the desired result from your decision is far more likely to occur.

Just as a pilot who does not calculate speeds before takeoff, anyone forming a habit who does not have a plan such as "Obstacle Avoidance Procedures" can end their habit of taking flight and therefore never experience transformation.

The best Obstacle Avoidance Procedures one can ever have are:

#1 – Relentless Preparation

#2 – Tracker Tools **(see THE FOLLOWING PAGE)**

#3 – Give Your Habit Time, 33 Days, 66 Days and 99 Days

#4 – Give Yourself Grace for Not Having a Perfect Takeoff

Most people hammer themselves when they screw up, and are self-destroying. It takes 66 days to form the habit, not 1 or 2 days, so give yourself some slack. You were not meant to form a habit in the first week. So relax when you screw up. People smoke for 5 years and then they expect to give everything up in the first day. Hey, you only have a limited amount of willpower and discipline. You are a human being, not a freaken machine. OK. Stop it.

The "tracker" is vital in forming a habit. A tracker is not just a system, but is a tool that releases emotion and monitors progress when your habit starts to take flight.

My Epoch Challenge
Habit Tracker

Habit: _____

99 Cruise	98	97	96	95	94	93
92	91	90	89	88	87	86
85	84	83	82	81	80	79
78	77	76	75	74	73	72
71	70	69	68	67		

Cruise Date: _____

66 Ascend	65	64	63	62	61	60
59	58	57	56	55	54	53
52	51	50	49	48	47	46
45	44	43	42	41	40	39
38	37	36	35	34		

Ascend Date: _____

33 Take Off	32	31	30	29	28	27
20	21	22	23	24	25	26
19	18	17	16	15	14	13
6	7	8	9	10	11	12
5	4	3	2	1		

Take Off Date: _____

Why do you want to complete the tracker? When you complete the tracker daily, there is an inner sense of accomplishment. Every day you complete a check mark, you feel that you have progressed. This becomes motivational. You will feel better and as we have discussed we make decisions based on logic yet we act on emotion. When our emotions are great, we take bigger steps forward. Also, if we slip up a day, our emotions help us to get back on track. Again remember that you were not meant to create the habit in the first week. So if you slip up, that is fine. The tracker helps you keep on track.

How to Complete the 99-Day Tracker

First, you can download a copy of the tracker at **MyEpochChallenge.com** You may decide to print the tracker.

On the tracker, write the Take Off date on the bottom of the tracker. Why do we work from the bottom up? Well, an aircraft starts on the runway and it goes up, just the way you are meant to go up. The first day of you starting to form your habit is your "Take Off "date.

Daily check off the box for that date. If you slip up, leave that day's box blank (empty).

When you get to day 33, you will see that things are getting easier.

Day 34 is your Ascend Date. This is when your habit starts to ascend.

Day 66 is when you start reaching your altitude and that is when your habit moves into a new phase of cruising, auto pilot where you will find that you will be using very little willpower and a lot less discipline to take the action you have wanted to. Your behavior begins to change drastically.

I would like to briefly reiterate what I have already said but in a slightly different way. Why? Because the foundation of forming habits is critical.

Preparation before day one of habit forming is critical. We need to understand that when changing a behavior, that we will not do it in 1 day. When we make a decision to do something, and the moments directly after the decision lack planning, preparation of tools and systems, the new decision will not take flight. Although decisions are powerful, decisions alone are not enough to sustain a transformation and to build a habit. Decisions are where new habits start, but just sitting in a cockpit of an aircraft without the aircraft moving will never get anyone to their destination. I believe in decisions, but decisions are not everything. They are part of the process, and one of many events.

If a pilot when entering the runway immediately pushes the power lever and throttle fully out, and then "pulls back" or rotates the rotator before the VR speed, the aircraft could, and probably would, lift too soon. Without enough lift under its wings, the aircraft is too heavy to take off and it would possibly crash. When we are forming habits, we must be careful not to assume we are already flying or our habits have taken off before they have been formed. This is a major reason why many people have resolutions that never happen. Many confidently speak out of their new behavior, new lifestyle, new resolution and new habit but lack what it takes to sustain flight.

When the Wright brothers experienced their first powered flight on December 17th, 1903 at Kitty Hawk, North Carolina, Orville Wright piloted the craft that stayed in the air 12 seconds and only flew 120 feet. That same day 3 additional flights were taken. Wilbur Wright piloted the record flight that day, which lasted 59 seconds and traveled 852 feet. They had been experimenting with flight from their bicycle shop since 1896 in Dayton, Ohio.

The Wright brothers had a spirit of relentless preparation. They had travelled to Kitty Hawk in 1902. They already had over 700 successful flights with their glider. They had to design their own engine that was light enough and powerful enough to support their flight. No auto manufacturer offered an engine like that. Only a decision to fly is not enough. The relentless preparation, continued planning, adjustments, and small action steps will lead us to our habits taking off.

What are you waiting for?

"Invigoration is what gets you moving. Habit is what keeps you moving."
– **Kurt Francis**

Afterword

Our futures are not really decided by us. Our habits are. The actions we take today change our tomorrow. We all tend to live by our past successes and past failures and not our imaginations, possibilities or potential. I have done many 99-day challenges and they have been remarkable.

I co-founded My Epoch Challenge, a 99-day program that helps one form habits. The program is designed to "transvigorate™" your life. It has helped many frustrated professionals who have had failed attempts to make long lasting changes in their lives. Those who have wanted to go to another level in their lives and careers but have not succeeded as they just did not know how to break through. This program has helped people in their careers who have lost their vision, lost their next step and lost their passion. We build our life by creating habit upon habit upon habit.

Recently I had the privilege of speaking at The Harvard Club of Boston. In the audience were 130 doctors, CEOs, lawyers, researchers, entrepreneurs and the world's best speakers. I shared a stage with Caitlyn Jenner and celebrity George

Ross. I was honored with a "Life Transformer" award because of my work and my passion on this subject. The outcome of My Epoch Challenge will invigorate your transformation that you have desired for your life. This program has touched many people across the globe. I would like to invite you set up a call with me on https://meetme.so/Kurt2 about My Epoch Challenge.

Here are what some have said about My Epoch Challenge:

Diane Schliep, Business Owner/Broker – "*I want to share with you that I have had a great experience with the Epoch Challenge. Kurt Francis was amazing with his ability to really take business to a different level than we were used to.*"

Brendan John – "*I just completed the Epoch Challenge with Kurt Francis and it's absolutely phenomenal. It's been worth every single second. The information and tools that I have received have really brought a whole sense of prosperity and accomplishment into my daily life. I gained a new sense of determination and drive, and believe that I can accomplish my dreams and the visions that I have in my life, which is so really exciting.*"

Made in the USA
Middletown, DE
03 December 2018